ADHD & the MODERN WOMAN:

Strategies for Managing Life's Demands

BRENDA MAYE

Table of Contents

Intro:

Attention Deficit Hyperactivity Disorder (ADHD) is a neurodevelopmental disorder that affects millions of individuals worldwide. Although ADHD is often associated with children, it is a lifelong condition that affects both men and women. The symptoms of ADHD, such as difficulty paying attention, impulsiveness, and hyperactivity, can create significant challenges in daily life and make it difficult to manage the demands of modern life.

Despite the prevalence of ADHD in the population, it is often misunderstood and stigmatized. Women with ADHD face unique challenges, as they may struggle to balance the demands of work, relationships, and home life. In addition, the symptoms of ADHD can often be misattributed to other causes, leading to misdiagnosis and a lack of proper treatment.

The purpose of "ADHD and the Modern Woman: Strategies for Managing Life's Demands" is to provide a comprehensive guide for women with ADHD.

The book aims to educate women about the nature of ADHD and to offer practical strategies for managing its symptoms and the demands of daily life.

This book provides a comprehensive overview of ADHD, including its causes, symptoms, and the impact it can have on different aspects of a woman's life. It also offers guidance on how to seek a proper diagnosis, as well as tips for managing symptoms and improving the overall quality of life.

One of the key themes of the book is the importance of self-care for women with ADHD. This includes developing coping mechanisms for dealing with stress, improving sleep habits, and taking time to recharge.

The book also provides advice on how to manage work-life balance and stay organized, including tips for prioritizing tasks, reducing distractions, and setting achievable goals.

In addition to practical strategies, the book includes a wealth of information on the latest research and treatments for ADHD. This includes an overview of the different types of medications and therapies used to treat ADHD, as well as information on alternative treatments, such as mindfulness and physical activity.

The book also provides guidance on how to navigate the healthcare system, including how to find a knowledgeable doctor and how to work with insurance companies.

In writing the book, the author draws on the experiences of real women with ADHD to provide a supportive and empathetic perspective.

Personal stories and testimonials offer insight into the challenges and triumphs of living with ADHD and provide inspiration for other women facing similar challenges.

In conclusion, "ADHD and the Modern Woman: Strategies for Managing Life's Demands" is a valuable resource for women with ADHD, their families, and healthcare professionals. It offers practical guidance and support for managing the demands of daily life, as well as the latest research and treatments for ADHD.

By educating women about ADHD and offering strategies for managing its symptoms, this book aims to empower women with ADHD to live their best lives and thrive in the modern world.

Chapter One: ADHD in women

Attention Deficit Hyperactivity Disorder (ADHD) is a neurodevelopmental disorder that affects individuals of all ages, including women. ADHD is characterized by inattention, hyperactivity, and impulsivity, and it can have a significant impact on a person's daily life and functioning.

While ADHD is often thought of as a condition that primarily affects children, many women are diagnosed with ADHD as adults. Women with ADHD may experience symptoms that are different from those seen in men, and their symptoms may be overlooked or misdiagnosed as a result.

Common symptoms of ADHD in women include:

Inattention: Women with ADHD may have difficulty paying attention, forgetfulness, disorganization, and distractions. They may also struggle with completing tasks, paying attention during conversations, or following through on commitments.

Hyperactivity: While hyperactivity is often associated with children with ADHD, some women with ADHD may also experience excessive restlessness or fidgeting.

Impulsivity: Women with ADHD may act without thinking and may have trouble controlling their impulses. This can result in impulsive spending, interrupting others, or acting on inappropriate or dangerous impulses.

Emotional dysregulation: Women with ADHD may experience mood swings, irritability, or emotional outbursts.

Time management difficulties: Women with ADHD may struggle with managing their time effectively and may have trouble meeting deadlines or completing tasks on time.

Executive dysfunction: Women with ADHD may have difficulties with planning, organizing, and executing tasks.

Diagnosis of ADHD in women can be challenging, as symptoms may be mistaken for other conditions, such as depression, anxiety, or menopause.

Women with ADHD may also experience a delay in diagnosis due to a lack of understanding of the disorder in women and the stigma associated with mental health conditions.

Treatment for ADHD in women typically involves a combination of medication and behavioral therapy. Medications such as stimulants or non-stimulants may be used to help manage symptoms of inattention, hyperactivity, and impulsivity. Behavioral therapy can help individuals with ADHD develop coping strategies, improve organization and time management skills, and manage stress.

It is important for women with ADHD to receive a proper diagnosis and treatment, as ADHD can have a significant impact on their daily lives. With the right support, women with ADHD can manage their symptoms and lead fulfilling, productive lives.

Symptoms, causes, and diagnosis

ADHD is a neurodevelopmental disorder that affects both men and women. However, ADHD in women often goes undiagnosed due to the fact that its symptoms in women maybe different from those in men and may not always fit the typical ADHD profile.

Here we will explore in detail the symptoms, causes, and diagnosis of ADHD in women.

Symptoms of ADHD in Women

Women with ADHD often exhibit a different set of symptoms compared to

men. While the symptoms of ADHD in men are often more hyperactive and impulsive, women with ADHD are more likely to experience symptoms that are predominantly inattentive. Common symptoms of ADHD in women include:

- Difficulty focusing or paying attention to tasks
- Poor organizational skills
- Procrastination
- Forgetfulness

- Difficulty following through with tasks and responsibilities
- Low self-esteem and self-confidence
- Difficulty with time management
- Chronic boredom
- Distracted easily
- Difficulty completing tasks
- Feelings of anxiety and depression

Causes of ADHD in Women

The exact cause of ADHD is unknown, but research suggests that it is a result of a combination of genetic, environmental, and neurological factors.

Some of the potential causes of ADHD in women include:

Genetics: ADHD tends to run in families and there is evidence that the disorder is partially inherited.

Brain Development: Studies have shown that individuals with ADHD have differences in the structure and function of certain areas of the brain compared to those without ADHD.

Environmental Factors: Exposure to toxins, such as lead, during pregnancy or childhood can increase the risk of developing ADHD.

Substance Abuse: Substance abuse during pregnancy can lead to ADHD in children.

Trauma: Children who experience traumatic events, such as abuse, neglect, or exposure to violence, are at an increased risk for developing ADHD.

Diagnosis of ADHD in Women

The diagnosis of ADHD in women can be difficult due to the fact that the symptoms in women often differ from those in men.

Additionally, the symptoms may be misinterpreted or dismissed as being due to other mental health conditions, such as anxiety or depression.

To diagnose ADHD, a healthcare provider will usually perform a comprehensive evaluation that includes a medical history, physical examination, and psychological testing.

Medical History: The healthcare provider will ask about the individual's symptoms, including when they started and how severe they are. They may also ask about the individual's family history of ADHD and other mental health conditions.

Physical Examination: The healthcare provider will perform a physical examination to rule out any medical conditions that may be causing the symptoms.

Psychological Testing: The healthcare provider may use psychological tests, such as the Conners' Adult ADHD Rating Scale or the Adult ADHD Self-Report Scale, to assess the individual's symptoms and determine if they meet the criteria for ADHD.

Generally, ADHD in women can be a complex and challenging disorder to diagnose. However, with the right evaluation and treatment, women with ADHD can lead fulfilling and productive lives. If you believe you may have ADHD, it is important to talk to a healthcare provider and get a proper evaluation and diagnosis.

Differences between ADHD in women and men

ADHD is a neurodevelopmental disorder that affects both men and women. However, there are some differences in the symptoms, presentation, and diagnosis of ADHD in men and women.

In men, ADHD is often diagnosed in childhood and is characterized by hyperactivity, impulsiveness, and inattention. Men with ADHD may have trouble sitting still, paying attention, and completing tasks. They may also struggle with managing their emotions and making decisions.

In women, ADHD is often not diagnosed until adulthood and is characterized by symptoms of inattention and forgetfulness.

Women with ADHD may have trouble organizing their thoughts, staying on task, and following through on responsibilities. They may also struggle with depression, anxiety, and low self-esteem.

It's important to note that these symptoms are not absolute and can vary greatly from person to person. Additionally, some studies have found that women with ADHD are less likely to receive a diagnosis, in part because they may exhibit symptoms that are different from what is traditionally considered "typical" for ADHD.

Overall, it's important for individuals who suspect they have ADHD to seek an evaluation from a healthcare professional, who can provide an accurate diagnosis and appropriate treatment.

Tips for managing symptoms & improving the overall quality of life

Here are some tips that may help women with ADHD manage their symptoms and improve their overall quality of life:

Create a routine: Having a structured routine can help women with ADHD stay organized and on track. This could involve making a daily to-do list, setting reminders, or using a planner.

Exercise regularly: Exercise has been shown to improve focus, concentration, and mood. Regular physical activity can also help reduce stress and increase overall well-being.

Get enough sleep: Sleep plays a crucial role in regulating mood and behavior. Women with ADHD should aim to get 7-9 hours of sleep each night to help manage their symptoms.

Minimize distractions: Distractions can be particularly challenging for women with ADHD, making it difficult to stay focused and on task. Minimizing distractions, such as turning off notifications on your phone or working in a quiet location can help improve focus and productivity.

Practice mindfulness: Mindfulness can help reduce stress and anxiety, and improve overall well-being. Activities such as meditation, deep breathing, and yoga can be helpful for women with ADHD.

Seek support: Women with ADHD may find it helpful to seek support from friends, family, or a therapist. Talking to someone about their symptoms and experiences can help reduce feelings of isolation and improve overall well-being.

Take medication as prescribed: For some women with ADHD, medication can be an effective way to manage symptoms. It's important to take medication as prescribed by a doctor and to regularly monitor any side effects.

It's also important to remember that everyone with ADHD is different, and what works for one person may not work for another. It may take some time and experimentation to find what works best, but with the right support and strategies, women with ADHD can lead fulfilling and successful lives.

a neurodevelopmental disorder characterized by symptoms such as inattention, hyperactivity, and impulsiveness.

In the workplace, women with ADHD may face several challenges, including difficulties with time management, organization, and prioritization. They may also struggle with maintaining focus and completing tasks, which can lead to stress and decreased productivity.

Additionally, women with ADHD may experience social difficulties, such as interpersonal conflicts and communication issues, which can affect their work relationships and professional reputation.

However, it's worth noting that everyone with ADHD experiences it differently, and some may have very mild symptoms that do not greatly impact their work, while others may struggle more. Also, some women with ADHD may have developed coping mechanisms to manage their symptoms and be successful in their careers.

Indeed, ADHD can affect the work of modern women, but with the right support and accommodations, many are able to overcome these challenges and succeed in their careers.

Effect on relationships

ADHD can impact relationships for individuals of all genders, including women. The symptoms of ADHD can make it difficult for individuals with the

condition to maintain focus, prioritize tasks, and manage time effectively, which can lead to problems in relationships.

For women with ADHD, some common relationship challenges may include:

Difficulty with communication: Women with ADHD may struggle to articulate their thoughts and feelings effectively, which can lead to misunderstandings and miscommunications with their partners.

Impulsiveness: Impulsiveness is a hallmark symptom of ADHD, and it can lead to impulsive behavior and decision-making in relationships. This can cause conflict and hurt feelings.

Disorganization: Women with ADHD may struggle with organizational skills, which can lead to forgetfulness, lateness, and disorganization in their relationships.

Distractibility: The distractibility that often accompanies ADHD can make it difficult for women with the condition to fully engage in their relationships, which can lead to feelings of disconnection and frustration.

It's important to note that while ADHD can present significant challenges in relationships, it is manageable with the right support and accommodations. Women with ADHD can work with their partners and healthcare providers to develop strategies for improving communication, managing impulsiveness, and staying organized, among other things.

Additionally, therapy and/or medication can be helpful for managing the symptoms of ADHD and improving functioning in relationships.

Effect on self-esteem

Effects on women's overall well-being
ADHD can have significant effects on the overall well-being of modern women. Women with ADHD often face challenges in their personal and professional lives, and these challenges can have a profound impact on their mental and physical health.

In terms of personal life, women with ADHD may struggle with time management and organization, leading to difficulties in completing tasks and meeting deadlines. This can cause feelings of stress, frustration, and low self-esteem.

Additionally, women with ADHD may experience relationship difficulties, including difficulties in communication and interpersonal dynamics.

In the professional realm, women with ADHD may face challenges in the workplace, such as difficulty with attention

to detail, difficulty in following through on tasks, and difficulty in prioritizing work responsibilities. These challenges can lead to decreased job performance and job satisfaction, and in some cases, unemployment.

Furthermore, women with ADHD may also experience physical health problems, such as fatigue, sleep disturbances, and decreased energy levels. This can lead to decreased physical activity, which can further impact overall well-being.

It's important to emphasize that with proper support and treatment, women with ADHD can lead fulfilling and successful lives.

Treatment options for ADHD may include medication, therapy, and lifestyle changes such as regular exercise and a balanced diet.

Additionally, support from friends, family, and a healthcare professional can be invaluable in managing symptoms and improving overall well-being.

Chapter Three: Strategies for managing time & organization

ADHD can be a challenging condition for women, especially when it comes to managing time and staying organized. Here are some strategies for managing time and organization for women with ADHD.

Make a list: Write down all the tasks you need to accomplish, along with deadlines and priorities. This helps you focus and remember what needs to be done, reducing stress and anxiety.

Use a planner: Keep a physical or digital planner to track your appointments, meetings, and to-do lists. This can help you stay on top of your schedule and avoid double-booking or missing important deadlines.

Break tasks into smaller steps: Large tasks can feel overwhelming, so breaking them down into smaller, manageable steps can help you stay focused and avoid procrastination.

Use reminders: Set reminders on your phone, or computer, or use a sticky note to remind you of upcoming deadlines and appointments.

Minimize distractions: Find a quiet and organized workspace to minimize distractions and maximize productivity. Consider using noise-canceling headphones to block out background noise.

Delegate: Don't be afraid to delegate tasks to others, especially if you feel overwhelmed. Delegating tasks can help you free up time to focus on other important tasks.

Prioritize self-care: Taking care of yourself is important for overall well-being and can help reduce stress and anxiety, which can make it easier to manage time and stay organized.

Seek support: Talk to friends, family, or a therapist about your ADHD and how it affects your daily life. They can offer support and help you develop strategies for managing time and staying organized.

Remember, managing time and staying organized with ADHD is a continuous process and it may take some time to find what works best for you. Be patient with yourself and don't be afraid to make adjustments as needed.

Mindfulness and self-care for women with ADHD

Mindfulness and self-care are important for everyone but can be especially beneficial for women with ADHD.

Here are some strategies for practicing mindfulness and self-care for women with ADHD:

Practice mindfulness meditation: Mindfulness meditation can help you focus your attention, reduce stress and anxiety, and improve your overall sense of well-being. Set aside a few minutes each day to simply sit and focus on your breath.

Exercise regularly: Regular exercise can help reduce symptoms of ADHD, improve focus and attention, and boost mood. Find an activity that you enjoy and make it a regular part of your routine.

Get enough sleep: Sleep is crucial for managing ADHD symptoms. Aim to get 7-9 hours of sleep each night and establish a regular sleep schedule.

Take breaks and have fun: Taking breaks and engaging in leisure activities can help reduce stress and improve your overall mood. Find activities that you enjoy and make time for them regularly.

Connect with others: Building strong social connections can provide support, reduce stress, and improve overall well-being. Make time for friends and family, or consider joining a support group for women with ADHD.

Practice self-compassion: Women with ADHD may experience negative self-talk and feelings of shame or guilt. It's important to practice self-compassion and remind yourself that you are doing the best you can.

Always remember, everyone's experience with ADHD is unique, and what works for one person may not work for another. It's important to be patient with yourself and try different strategies until you find what works best for you.

Tips for prioritizing tasks, reducing distractions, and setting achievable goals

Here are some tips that can help prioritize tasks, reduce distractions, and set achievable goals:

Make a to-do list: Write down all your tasks for the day and prioritize them in order of importance. This helps you stay focused on what needs to be done and reduces the chances of getting overwhelmed.

Minimize distractions: Identify the distractions that are preventing you from completing your tasks and find ways to eliminate them. For example, you can turn off notifications on your phone, use noise-canceling headphones or work in a quiet space.

Set achievable goals: Break larger tasks into smaller, manageable steps and set realistic deadlines for each step. This makes it easier to stay on track and avoid feeling overwhelmed.

Use reminders: Use reminders to keep yourself on track and avoid forgetting important tasks. You can use a physical planner, a digital calendar, or a task management app to set reminders.

Take breaks: It's important to take breaks and give your brain a rest. You can take a walk, do some stretching, or engage in a hobby to help recharge your batteries.

Practice self-care: Taking care of yourself is important for managing ADHD symptoms.

Try to get enough sleep, eat a healthy diet, and engage in physical activity regularly.

Seek support: Don't be afraid to seek help from family, friends, or a mental health professional. Having a support system can make a big difference in managing ADHD symptoms.

Remember, everyone with ADHD is unique, and what works for one person may not work for another. It may take some trial and error to find the strategies that work best for you, but with patience and persistence, you can manage your symptoms and achieve your goals.

Chapter 4: Role of medication in managing ADHD symptoms in modern women

ADHD is a neurodevelopmental disorder that affects both men and women, but the symptoms, as we've learned, can manifest differently in women as compared to men.

As stated earlier in this book, women with ADHD often experience symptoms like forgetfulness, disorganization, low self-esteem, and depression, which can result in difficulties in daily life activities.

The conventional treatments for ADHD include medication, psychotherapy, and lifestyle changes, with medication being the most commonly used. Hence, we will discuss the role of medication in managing ADHD symptoms in women.

Medication plays a crucial role in managing ADHD symptoms in women by reducing hyperactivity, impulsiveness, and improving attention and focus.

The most commonly prescribed medications for ADHD are stimulants such as Methylphenidate (Ritalin, Concerta), Amphetamines (Adderall, Vyvanse,) and non-stimulant medications such as Atomoxetine (Strattera). These medications increase the levels of neurotransmitters like dopamine and norepinephrine in the brain, which are responsible for regulating attention and impulse control.

Stimulant medications, such as Methylphenidate and Amphetamines, are considered first-line treatments for ADHD. They are effective in reducing hyperactivity and impulsiveness, and improving attention and focus. They have been extensively researched and have a well-established safety profile when taken as prescribed.

Women with ADHD who take stimulant medications report improvements in their daily life activities such as increased productivity, better organizational skills, and improved relationships.

However, stimulant medications have some side effects, including decreased appetite, weight loss, and trouble sleeping. Women with ADHD who have a history of substance abuse or addiction may not be suitable candidates for stimulant medications, as they have a high potential for abuse. Therefore, it is crucial to assess the risk-benefit ratio of stimulant medications before starting treatment and to monitor the women carefully while they are on the medication.

Non-stimulant medications, such as Atomoxetine, are another option for managing ADHD symptoms in women. They are considered a second-line treatment option and are used when stimulant medications are not suitable or when women do not respond to stimulants.

Non-stimulant medications work by increasing the levels of norepinephrine in the brain, which is responsible for regulating attention and impulse control. Non-stimulant medications are effective in reducing hyperactivity and impulsiveness and improving attention and focus.

Atomoxetine has a lower potential for abuse compared to stimulant medications and is considered safe for women with ADHD. However, it can cause side effects such as decreased appetite, weight loss, and nausea, and it may take several weeks to start working. Women who have liver problems or are taking other medications that interact with Atomoxetine may not be suitable candidates for this medication.

Truly, medication plays a crucial role in managing ADHD symptoms in women. Stimulant medications and non-stimulant medications have been found to be effective in reducing hyperactivity and impulsiveness and improving attention and focus.

Women who are considering medication for ADHD should discuss the options and their potential side effects with their healthcare provider to determine the best course of treatment.

Lifestyle changes and psychotherapy can also be effective in managing ADHD symptoms and should be used in combination with medication for maximum benefit.

It is essential to monitor women carefully while they are on medication and to adjust the dosage as needed to ensure that they are receiving the most benefits with the least amount of side effects.

Benefits and potential side effects of using medication to manage ADHD symptoms in women

Medication is one of the most commonly used treatments for ADHD in women, and has been shown to be effective in reducing the symptoms of inattention, impulsivity, and hyperactivity.

The benefits of using medication to manage ADHD symptoms in women include:

Improved focus and attention: ADHD medications can help improve focus, concentration, and attention, allowing women with ADHD to better complete tasks and pay attention in meetings, lectures, and other situations.

Increased productivity: By reducing symptoms of ADHD, women may find that they are able to be more productive and efficient in their daily lives.

Improved relationships: Women with ADHD may find that their relationships with family, friends, and coworkers improve as a result of their increased ability to focus and control impulsive behavior.

Reduced stress: Women with ADHD often experience high levels of stress and anxiety, and medication can help to reduce these symptoms, leading to improved overall well-being.

However, like all medications, there are potential side effects associated with the use of ADHD medications in women:

Insomnia: Some women may experience difficulty sleeping after taking ADHD medications, which can lead to feelings of fatigue during the day.

Loss of appetite: Some women may experience a decrease in appetite after starting ADHD medication, which can lead to weight loss.

Nervousness: Some women may feel nervous or jittery after taking ADHD medications, especially if they take the medication on an empty stomach.

Cardiac problems: There have been rare cases of cardiac problems associated with the use of ADHD medications, particularly in women with pre-existing heart conditions.

Mood changes: ADHD medications can sometimes affect mood and lead to feelings of anxiety, depression, or irritability.

It's important to remember that not all women with ADHD will experience side effects and that the benefits of medication often outweigh the potential risks. It's also important to work closely with a healthcare provider to monitor the effects of medication and to adjust the dose as needed.

Importance of working with a healthcare provider

Finding the right medication and dose to manage ADHD symptoms can be a complex process and it is important to work closely with a healthcare provider. This is because everyone with ADHD is unique and may respond differently to different medications and doses.

The following are some reasons why working with a healthcare provider is important when using medication to manage ADHD symptoms:

Proper Diagnosis: A healthcare provider can diagnose ADHD and rule out other potential causes of symptoms, such as sleep disorders, anxiety, or depression.

Individualized Treatment Plan: A healthcare provider can help develop a personalized treatment plan based on the specific needs and symptoms of the individual, taking into account their medical history, lifestyle, and other factors.

Monitoring for Side Effects: A healthcare provider can monitor for side effects and adjust the dose as needed to minimize them. They can also monitor for any interactions between ADHD medication and other medications the individual may be taking.

Safety: A healthcare provider can ensure that the individual is taking the medication safely and in the proper dose. They can also monitor for any underlying medical conditions that may affect the individual's ability to take ADHD medication.

Long-Term Management: A healthcare provider can help manage the long-term use of ADHD medication, including monitoring for effectiveness and adjusting the dose as needed over time.

In summary, working with a healthcare provider is crucial when using medication to manage ADHD symptoms. They can help ensure that the individual is taking the medication safely and effectively and that they receive the best possible care.

The role of medication in combination with other treatments to manage ADHD in women

The use of medication in combination with other treatments is a common approach to managing ADHD in women.

Medications used to treat ADHD include stimulants, such as methylphenidate (Ritalin, Concerta) and amphetamines (Adderall), as well as non-stimulant medications, such as atomoxetine (Strattera). These medications help to regulate brain chemicals, improve attention, and reduce hyperactivity and impulsiveness.

However, medication alone may not be enough to effectively manage ADHD in women. Research has shown that a comprehensive approach to treatment that includes medication, psychotherapy, and lifestyle changes can be more effective in managing the symptoms of ADHD in women.

Psychotherapy, such as cognitive behavioral therapy, can help women with ADHD learn new coping skills and manage the challenges of daily life.

Additionally, lifestyle changes, such as creating a structured environment, reducing stress, and maintaining a healthy diet and exercise regimen, can help to mitigate the symptoms of ADHD.

It is important to work with a healthcare provider who is knowledgeable about ADHD in women to develop a personalized treatment plan. The goal of treatment should be to help women with ADHD manage their symptoms, improve their quality of life, and achieve their personal and professional goals.

Challenges women with ADHD may face in accessing and affording medications

Women with ADHD often face several challenges in accessing and affording medications. Some of these challenges include:

Diagnosis: Women with ADHD are often misdiagnosed or underdiagnosed, leading to a delay in accessing appropriate treatment and medication. This can be due to the stereotype that ADHD is a disorder that primarily affects boys and men.

Cost: ADHD medications can be expensive, and many women with ADHD struggle to afford them. This is especially true for those who are uninsured or underinsured.

Stigma: There is still a significant amount of stigma surrounding mental health conditions, including ADHD. This can lead to reluctance on the part of some women to seek treatment and medication, for fear of being labeled as "crazy" or "weak".

Lack of information: Many women with ADHD may not have access to accurate information about the condition and its treatments. This can result in confusion and uncertainty about what medications are available, what they do, and how to access them.

Challenges with accessing healthcare: Some women with ADHD may have difficulty accessing healthcare services due to geographic, financial, or other barriers. For example, they may live in rural areas without access to specialized ADHD clinics, or they may be unable to take time off work to attend appointments.

To address these challenges, it is important to provide women with ADHD with accurate information about the condition and its treatments, to increase public awareness and reduce stigma, and to make sure that affordable treatment options are available to those who need them. This can involve advocating for policies that make ADHD medications more accessible and affordable and working with healthcare providers to ensure that they are knowledgeable about the unique needs of women with ADHD.

The importance of ongoing monitoring and reassessment of ADHD symptoms and medication effectiveness

The importance of ongoing monitoring and reassessment of ADHD symptoms and medication effectiveness cannot be overstated. Attention Deficit Hyperactivity Disorder (ADHD) is a chronic condition that often requires ongoing treatment and management, and regular monitoring and reassessment can help ensure that the individual's treatment plan remains effective over time.

For individuals taking medication for ADHD, it is important to regularly monitor the effectiveness of the medication, including any side effects or changes in symptoms. The individual's response to medication can change over time, and medication that was once effective may no longer be providing the same level of relief. Regular monitoring allows the healthcare provider to adjust the dosage, switch to a different medication, or consider alternative treatment options if needed.

In addition to monitoring the effectiveness of the medication, it is also important to regularly assess the individual's ADHD symptoms. As individuals age, their symptoms may change, and it is essential to ensure that the treatment plan remains effective in addressing their current symptoms.

Additionally, individuals with ADHD may experience comorbid conditions, such as anxiety or depression, that can impact their symptoms and treatment plan. Regular reassessment can help identify these changes and ensure that the individual is receiving the appropriate care and support.

Overall, ongoing monitoring and reassessment of ADHD symptoms and medication effectiveness are crucial to ensuring that individuals with ADHD receive the best possible care and support in managing their condition.

Women with ADHD who prefer not to use medication

For women who cannot or prefer not to use medication for ADHD, there are alternative treatments that can be considered. These include:

Psychotherapy: This type of therapy can help individuals with ADHD manage their symptoms, improve their relationships, and enhance their quality of life. Therapy can also help women with ADHD understand their condition and learn coping strategies.

Cognitive Behavioral Therapy (CBT): CBT can help individuals with ADHD identify and change negative thought patterns and behaviors that contribute to their symptoms. This type of therapy can also help individuals develop better organizational skills, manage time more effectively, and improve their ability to focus.

Mindfulness-based approaches: Mindfulness practices such as meditation, yoga, and tai chi can help individuals with ADHD reduce stress and improve focus and attention.

Lifestyle changes: Making changes to one's diet, exercise, and sleep patterns can help improve symptoms of ADHD. A healthy diet, regular exercise, and sufficient sleep can help regulate the body and mind, and reduce symptoms of ADHD.

Coaching and support groups: ADHD coaching can help individuals with ADHD develop and implement strategies for managing their symptoms. Support groups can also provide a sense of community and a place for individuals with ADHD to connect with others who understand their experiences.

It is important to remember that each person with ADHD is unique and what works for one person may not work for another. It is also important to work with a mental health professional to find the best treatment approach for your individual needs.

Current research and trends in the use of medication to manage ADHD symptoms in women

The use of medication to manage ADHD symptoms in women has been the subject of much research over the years, and the current trends suggest that it is an effective option for many women with ADHD.

The most commonly used medications for ADHD are stimulants, such as methylphenidate (Ritalin, Concerta) and amphetamines (Adderall, Dexedrine), which have been shown to be effective in improving symptoms of inattention, impulsiveness, and hyperactivity in both men and women with ADHD.

However, research has also shown that there may be some differences in the way that ADHD medications affect women compared to men. For example, studies have shown that women may be more sensitive to the side effects of stimulant medications, such as decreased appetite, weight loss, and sleep disturbances.

Additionally, women with ADHD may respond differently to different types of medication and may require lower doses or different formulations of medication to achieve optimal symptom control.

It is also important to note that medication is not the only option for managing ADHD symptoms in women. In addition to medication, behavioral therapies, such as cognitive behavioral therapy and mindfulness-based approaches, have also been shown to be effective in managing ADHD symptoms in women. Some women may also find that lifestyle changes, such as regular exercise, a healthy diet, and good sleep habits, can help to manage their symptoms.

While the use of medication is a common and effective option for managing ADHD symptoms in women, it is important to consider individual differences and to work with a healthcare provider to determine the best treatment plan.

Additionally, a combination of medication and other strategies, such as therapy and lifestyle changes, maybe the most effective approach for many women with ADHD.

The role of therapy and counseling in managing ADHD and improving mental health

Therapy and counseling play a significant role in managing ADHD.

Therapy can help individuals with ADHD develop coping strategies and improve their executive functioning skills, such as organization and time management. For example, cognitive-behavioral therapy (CBT) can help individuals identify and change negative thought patterns, and improve their self-esteem and resilience.

Counseling can also help individuals with ADHD address any comorbid conditions, such as depression, anxiety, or substance abuse. Additionally, counseling can provide a supportive environment for individuals to discuss the challenges they face and learn new coping mechanisms. Family therapy can also be beneficial in addressing any issues within the family dynamic that may be affecting the individual with ADHD.

Therapy and counseling are effective tools in the management of ADHD and the improvement of mental health. They can help individuals with ADHD better understand their condition, develop coping strategies, and improve their overall well-being.

Therapy for women with ADHD

There is no one-size-fits-all answer to particular therapy women with ADHD should use as the effectiveness of therapy can vary greatly depending on the individual and their specific needs and circumstances. However, some of the most commonly used and evidence-based therapies for women with ADHD include:

Cognitive-behavioral therapy (CBT): This is a common form of therapy for ADHD. This type of therapy helps individuals identify and change negative thought patterns and behaviors that contribute to their symptoms. It can also teach coping skills, such as time management, organization, and goal setting.

Mindfulness-based therapy: This therapy helps individuals with ADHD become more aware of their thoughts and behaviors in the present moment, and develop strategies for managing symptoms.

Behavioral therapy: Specifically parent- or teacher-led training, behavioral therapy can also be effective in managing ADHD symptoms. This type of therapy focuses on improving specific behaviors and provides strategies for managing challenging behaviors.

Coaching: This type of therapy involves working with a coach to develop personalized strategies for managing symptoms, such as time management and organization skills.

Psychotherapy: This type of therapy can help individuals with ADHD address any co-occurring mental health conditions and develop coping strategies for their ADHD symptoms.

Family therapy: In addition to individual therapy, family therapy can also be helpful for individuals with ADHD and their families. Family therapy can provide support, education, and help improve communication and relationships within the family.

It's important to note that medications, such as stimulants and non-stimulants, are also often used to treat ADHD in women. The most effective treatment plan will depend on the individual's specific needs and preferences. It is recommended to work with a mental health professional or physician to develop a personalized treatment plan.

Overall, therapy can be a valuable tool in the management of ADHD and can help individuals lead fulfilling and productive lives.

Strategies for counseling women with ADHD

Counseling can be a beneficial option for women with ADHD who are looking for support and guidance. A trained therapist can help women with ADHD understand and manage their symptoms, improve their relationships, and develop coping strategies for the challenges they face.

In counseling, women with ADHD can learn about the impact of ADHD on their daily lives and develop strategies for organization, time management, and goal setting. They can also work on building self-esteem, managing stress and anxiety, and improving communication skills.

Some strategies for counseling women with ADHD include:

Understanding the unique challenges: Women with ADHD often face challenges that are different from men, such as lower levels of diagnosis, more difficulty with inattention than hyperactivity, and higher levels of anxiety and depression. Counselors should take these differences into account when working with women with ADHD.

Emphasizing strengths: Women with ADHD have unique strengths and talents, such as creativity, intuition, and empathy. Counselors can help women with ADHD identify and build on these strengths.

Improving organizational skills: Women with ADHD often struggle with organization and time management. Counselors can teach women with ADHD practical strategies for improving these skills, such as using a planner, breaking tasks into smaller steps, and prioritizing.

Addressing anxiety and depression: Women with ADHD are more likely to experience anxiety and depression. Counselors should address these co-occurring conditions and provide support and coping strategies.

Encouraging self-care: Women with ADHD often struggle with self-care and taking care of themselves. Counselors can help women with ADHD develop a self-care routine that includes exercise, healthy eating, and stress management techniques.

Providing support for relationships: Women with ADHD often face challenges in their relationships, such as communication difficulties, impulsiveness, and forgetfulness. Counselors can provide support and strategies for improving communication and strengthening relationships.

It's important to remember that each woman with ADHD is unique, and the counseling approach should be tailored to meet her specific needs and goals.

Guidance on how to navigate the healthcare system

Navigating the healthcare system can be challenging for anyone, but it can be especially difficult for women with ADHD. Here are some tips to help you navigate the healthcare system effectively:

Find a doctor who specializes in ADHD: Look for a doctor who has experience in treating ADHD and is knowledgeable about the condition. Ask for recommendations from friends, family, or support groups.

Educate yourself about ADHD: The more you know about ADHD, the better equipped you will be to make informed decisions about your treatment. Read up on the latest research and treatments, and bring this information to your doctor.

Be open and honest with your doctor: Don't be afraid to discuss your symptoms, concerns, and experiences with your doctor. The more information you provide, the better your doctor will be able to understand your situation and provide the right treatment.

Keep a record of your symptoms and treatments: Write down your symptoms and the treatments you have tried. This will help you keep track of what is working and what isn't, and will also be helpful for your doctor.

Be proactive: Don't wait for your doctor to bring up important topics. If you have concerns or questions, bring them up during your appointment.

Advocate for yourself: Don't be afraid to ask for what you need. If you feel like your doctor is not listening to you or taking your symptoms seriously, consider finding a different doctor.

Consider therapy: Cognitive behavioral therapy (CBT) and other forms of therapy can be helpful for managing ADHD symptoms. Ask your doctor for recommendations on therapists who specialize in ADHD.

Seek support from others: Joining a support group for women with ADHD can be a great way to connect with others who are going through similar experiences. You can also seek support from friends, family, or a mental health professional.

By taking these steps and being proactive about your treatment, you can effectively navigate the healthcare system and receive the support you need to manage your ADHD symptoms.

How to find a knowledgeable doctor

Finding a knowledgeable doctor for attention deficit hyperactivity disorder can be a challenge, but it's important to find a healthcare provider who is well-informed about the condition and can provide you with effective treatment.

Here are some tips that might help:

Ask for recommendations: Reach out to friends, family, or support groups for recommendations on doctors who have a good reputation for treating ADHD.

Research providers online: Look for doctors who specialize in treating ADHD. Websites such as Healthgrades, Vitals, and ZocDoc can be helpful for finding healthcare providers and reading patient reviews.

Look for a doctor with experience: Consider a doctor who has a substantial amount of experience in diagnosing and treating ADHD. Ask the doctor how many patients with ADHD they see in a year.

Consider the type of doctor: There are several types of healthcare providers who can diagnose and treat ADHD, including pediatricians, family medicine doctors, psychiatrists, and neurologists. Consider seeing a specialist who has experience with ADHD.

Ask about their approach to treatment: It's important to find a doctor who supports your treatment goals and is open to working with you to find the best approach for your needs.

Schedule an appointment: Schedule an appointment with the doctor to see if you feel comfortable with them and if they are knowledgeable about ADHD.

Remember, finding the right doctor is a process, and it may take some time. But taking the time to find the right healthcare provider can make a significant difference in the quality of care you receive for your ADHD.

How to work with insurance companies

Working with insurance companies can be a challenging process, particularly when it comes to getting coverage for ADHD treatment.

Here are some steps you can take to make the process smoother:

Know your insurance policy: Before you start working with an insurance company, take the time to fully understand your policy and what it covers. This can help you avoid any surprises down the line.

Build a strong case: Insurance companies will often require documentation from your doctor, such as a diagnosis, treatment plan, and progress notes, in order to approve coverage for ADHD treatment.

Make sure you have all of this information on hand and that it is well-organized and easy for the insurance company to understand.

Be persistent: Don't give up if your first claim is denied. Many insurance companies will require you to appeal the decision and provide additional information before they will approve coverage. Be prepared to follow up multiple times and provide all the information they request.

Seek out advocacy groups: There are many organizations and support groups that can help you navigate the insurance process and advocate for the coverage you need. Consider reaching out to local or national advocacy groups for assistance.

Find out if medication is covered: ADHD medication can be expensive, but many insurance plans will cover the cost. If you're having trouble getting coverage for medication, consider asking your doctor for a generic alternative or for assistance with finding a patient assistance program.

Remember, working with insurance companies can be a time-consuming and complex process, but with persistence and patience, you can get the coverage you need for your ADHD treatment.

Chapter Five: Building a support network

Building a support network can be incredibly beneficial for women with ADHD, and can help in managing the symptoms and challenges associated with the condition. Here are a few steps you can take to build a support network:

Reach out to friends and family members: Talk to your loved ones about your ADHD and how it affects you. Explain what kind of support you need from them, whether it be just a listening ear or practical help with daily tasks.

Identify your needs: Take some time to think about what kind of support you need from others. Do you need someone to listen to you, help you with organization and time management, or offer encouragement and motivation?

Connect with other women with ADHD: Join support groups or online forums where you can connect with other women who understand what you're going through. This can be a great source of support, and you may even make new friends.

Work with a healthcare professional: A doctor or therapist who specializes in ADHD can be a valuable member of your support network. They can help you manage your symptoms, provide you with resources, and connect you with additional support.

Seek accommodations at work: If your ADHD is affecting your work performance, consider discussing accommodations with your employer. This could include a more flexible schedule, a quieter workspace, or modifications to your job duties.

Be proactive about self-care: Taking care of your physical and emotional well-being is important for managing ADHD symptoms. Engage in activities that bring you joy, such as exercise, hobbies, or spending time with loved ones.

Take advantage of resources: There are many resources available to help women with ADHD, including books, and websites. Take advantage of these resources to learn more about the condition and to find additional support.

Remember, building a support network takes time and effort, but it can make a big difference in helping you manage your ADHD. Be patient and don't be afraid to reach out for help when you need it.

My encounter with Lucia Jeffers, a woman with ADHD, might help you.

I met Lucia, a businesswoman, while I was conducting research for this book.

A friend of mine had told me about her and how she was doing well in her career despite her struggles with ADHD. I was eager to learn more about her story and reached out to her for an interview.

When I first met her, I was struck by her energy and enthusiasm. Despite her busy schedule, she was eager to share her experiences and insights with me. As she began to talk, she opened up about her struggles with ADHD and how she had built a support network of friends, family, and healthcare professionals to help her cope.

She told me that when she was first diagnosed with ADHD, she felt overwhelmed and unsure of how to manage her symptoms. However, with the help of her support network, she was able to develop strategies for staying organized, staying focused, and managing her time effectively.

One of the most important things she told me was the importance of open and honest communication with her loved ones and the healthcare team. She said that by sharing her struggles and working together, she was able to build a network of people who understood her needs and could support her in overcoming her challenges.

She also spoke about the various tools and strategies she used to manage her ADHD, such as medication, therapy, and mindfulness exercises. She told me that it was a constant process of experimentation and adjustment, but with the help of her support network, she was able to find the right balance that worked for her.

As she shared her story with me, I was inspired by her resilience and determination. Despite the challenges she faced, she had built a life for herself that was full of purpose and success. She was a true testament to the power of support and perseverance.

By the end of our conversation, I was filled with a newfound appreciation for the experiences of individuals with ADHD and the importance of support in overcoming challenges.

Lucia had built a support network that was helping her to thrive, and I left our conversation feeling grateful for the opportunity to learn from her story.

The story of Lucia should motivate any woman with ADHD. Whether it's friends, family, or healthcare professionals, having people in your corner who understand and support you can make all the difference.

Lucia told me that her friends have been a constant source of encouragement and understanding.

"They listen when I need to vent about the difficulties I face," she said, "and they celebrate with me when I have successes, no matter how small they may be."

"My family has also been a key component of my support network. They may not fully understand what it's like to have ADHD, but they love and support me unconditionally. Having their backing has given me the confidence to keep pushing forward, even on my toughest days.

"In addition to my loved ones, I've also found great support from healthcare professionals. Whether it's my therapist, who helps me work through my emotions, or my doctor, who works with me to manage my symptoms, they have been invaluable in helping me navigate the challenges of ADHD."

Though having a support network doesn't make the challenges of ADHD disappear, it, however, does make them more manageable. So, if you're feeling overwhelmed or alone, I encourage you to reach out to those around you. You don't have to face this journey alone.

Remember, as a woman with ADHD, you are strong, capable, and worthy of love and support. And with the right people by your side, you can overcome anything.

Chapter six: Finding the right balance between work $ personal life for modern women with ADHD

Finding the right balance between work and personal life can be a challenge for anyone, but it can be especially challenging for women with ADHD.

ADHD can cause difficulties with time management, organization, and impulse control, which can make it difficult to effectively balance work and personal responsibilities.

However, there are strategies that can help:

Create a schedule: Creating a schedule can help you stay on track and manage your time more effectively. This can include time for work tasks, personal responsibilities, and self-care activities.

Use a to-do list: A to-do list can help you keep track of tasks and prioritize what needs to be done first.

Minimize distractions: Distractions can be especially challenging for individuals with ADHD. Try to minimize distractions at work by closing your office door, using noise-canceling headphones, or working in a quiet location.

Set boundaries: It's important to set boundaries between work and personal life to avoid burnout. Make sure to set aside time for family, friends, and hobbies outside of work hours.

Consider medication: If your ADHD is affecting your ability to balance work and personal life, medication can be helpful. Talk to your doctor about whether medication might be right for you.

Seek support: Finally, it's important to seek support from family, friends, and colleagues. This can help you feel more supported and less isolated, and can provide you with the resources you need to succeed.

Always remember, everyone's experience with ADHD is different, and what works for one person may not work for another. It may take some time to find the right balance, but with the right strategies and support, it is possible.

Chapter Seven: Dealing with the stigma associated with ADHD & advocating for oneself

ADHD affects millions of people worldwide. Despite its prevalence, many individuals with ADHD still face stigma and misunderstandings about the condition. This stigma can come from friends, family members, coworkers, and even healthcare professionals, which can make it difficult for people with ADHD to advocate for themselves and receive the support and resources they need.

Here are some ways to deal with the stigma associated with ADHD and advocate for oneself:

Educate Yourself: Gain a deep understanding of ADHD, including its causes, symptoms, and treatments. This will help you feel more confident and equipped to answer questions and correct misunderstandings about the condition.

Connect with Others: Joining a support group for individuals with ADHD can provide a sense of community and help reduce feelings of isolation. Sharing experiences and learning from others can also provide valuable insights and coping strategies.

Be Open and Honest: Don't be afraid to talk about your experience with ADHD, including the challenges and successes. This can help others see the condition in a more positive light and dispel misconceptions.

Seek Professional Support: Work with a healthcare professional who is knowledgeable about ADHD and can provide an accurate diagnosis and effective treatment plan. This can also help you feel more confident and empowered when advocating for yourself.

Speak Up: If you feel like someone is not treating you with the respect you deserve or you are not receiving the support you need, it is important to speak up. This could mean having a conversation with a friend or family member, or requesting accommodations in the workplace.

Practice Self-Care: Taking care of yourself, including getting enough sleep, exercising, and engaging in activities that bring you joy, can help boost your mood and give you the energy to advocate for yourself.

By understanding and embracing your ADHD, connecting with others, seeking professional support, and speaking up, you can help break down the stigma associated with the condition and advocate for yourself effectively.

Remember, it is important to be kind and compassionate with yourself, and to seek help and support when needed.

Chapter Eight: The importance of setting realistic goals and managing expectations

It is indeed crucial for women with ADHD to set realistic goals and manage their expectations.

ADHD can lead to difficulties with planning, organization, and impulse control, which can negatively impact one's daily life and relationships, however, setting achievable goals and managing expectations can help reduce stress, improve confidence, and increase success.

Here are some tips for setting realistic goals and managing expectations for women with ADHD:

Break down larger goals into smaller, manageable tasks: This can help reduce feelings of overwhelm and increase the likelihood of success.

Prioritize tasks based on importance and urgency: Focus on what needs to be done first and what can wait. This can help ensure that you are making progress on the most important tasks.

Use a planner or to-do list: Writing down tasks and deadlines can help you keep track of what needs to be done and avoid forgetting important tasks.

Be flexible: Life is unpredictable and things do not always go as planned. It's important to be open to adjusting your goals and expectations as needed.

Celebrate your successes: Recognizing your accomplishments, no matter how small, can help boost your confidence and motivation to keep working towards your goals.

Seek support: Having someone to talk to, whether a friend, family member, or professional, can provide valuable perspective and help you manage your expectations.

It's important to remember that everyone's experience with ADHD is unique and what works for one person may not work for another. It's okay to experiment and find what strategies work best for you.

Chapter Nine: Draw inspiration from successful public figures with ADHD

There are many successful public figures with ADHD who serve as great inspirations for women with ADHD. Here are a few examples:

Howie Mandel: Although Howie Mandel is a male public figure, he has been open about his ADHD and how it has impacted his life and career. He uses medication to manage his symptoms and also practices mindfulness, exercise, and stress management techniques to stay focused and calm.

Mandel, a well-known comedian, actor, and television host, has spoken about his experiences in interviews, on television shows, and in his book "Here's the Deal: Don't Touch Me."

In these appearances, Mandel has talked about how his ADHD affects his daily life, how he has learned to manage it, and how it has influenced his career. He has also spoken about how he has used his experiences with ADHD and OCD to help others who are struggling with similar issues.

Overall, Mandel has been a strong advocate for raising awareness about ADHD and mental health, and he has encouraged others to seek help if they are struggling with similar issues.

Michael Phelps: The retired American Olympic swimmer, has spoken openly about his struggles with ADHD.

He was diagnosed with ADHD when he was 9 years old, and he has said that it has affected many aspects of his life, including his school work and early swimming career. However, Phelps has also credited his success in swimming, including his record-breaking number of Olympic medals, to his ADHD. He has said that his ADHD gave him a unique ability to focus and visualize his races, which helped him to perform at the highest level.

Tyra Banks: The former supermodel and current talk show host, has been open about her experiences with ADHD. In interviews and on her talk show, she has discussed how ADHD has affected her life and her career.

Banks has said that she was diagnosed with ADHD as a child and that it has often made it difficult for her to focus and stay organized.

However, she has also talked about how she has learned to manage her ADHD symptoms through various strategies, such as therapy, medication, and mindfulness practices.

Banks has used her platform to raise awareness about ADHD and to encourage others who may be struggling with the condition to seek help and support. She has encouraged people to talk openly about mental health and to remove the stigma surrounding conditions like ADHD.

By sharing her own experiences, Banks hopes to help others feel less alone and more empowered to take control of their own mental health.

Ricki Lake: An American actress, television host, and producer, Ricki Lake has been open about her struggles with ADHD.

She has stated that she was diagnosed with ADHD in her late 30s, and that it was a huge relief to finally understand the reason behind her difficulties with focus, organization, and impulsiveness.

In interviews and public appearances, Lake has spoken about the challenges of living with ADHD and the impact it has had on her life and career. She has also been a strong advocate for raising awareness about ADHD and destigmatizing mental health conditions.

Additionally, Lake has stated that medication has been a helpful tool for managing her ADHD symptoms, but she also believes in the importance of incorporating other strategies, such as therapy and mindfulness, into her overall wellness routine.

Overall, Ricki Lake's openness about her ADHD diagnosis has helped to raise awareness about the condition and encouraged others to seek support and treatment if they think they might have ADHD.

Ty Pennington: The TV host and carpenter, has spoken publicly about his experience with attention deficit hyperactivity disorder. In interviews, he shared that he was diagnosed with ADHD in his early 30s and that it was a challenging realization.

He has also discussed how he's learned to manage his symptoms with medication and therapy.

Pennington has been open about the difficulties he faced in his personal and professional life because of his ADHD, and how he's worked to overcome them.

He has talked about the stigma surrounding ADHD and how he wants to raise awareness about the condition and help others who may be struggling with it.

He has said that while having ADHD can be challenging, it can also be a strength and that he's learned to channel his energy and creativity in positive ways.

Channing Tatum: Actor and dancer, best known for his roles in "Step Up" and "Magic Mike," has been open about his experience with ADHD.

In an interview, he mentioned that he was diagnosed with ADHD when he was a child and that it has affected his life in various ways. He has described himself as someone who has trouble sitting still and staying focused on one task for a long time, which are common symptoms of ADHD.

Tatum has also mentioned that he has learned to manage his ADHD through various techniques such as meditation and exercise.

Additionally, Tatum has spoken about how his ADHD made him feel different and isolated when he was growing up, but that it has also given him a unique perspective and energy that has helped him in his career as an actor.

He has encouraged others who have ADHD to embrace their differences and not be afraid to seek help in managing their symptoms.

Simone Biles: The Olympic gymnast has spoken publicly about being diagnosed with ADHD. In a 2018 interview, she said that she was diagnosed with ADHD when she was a child and that it was a challenge for her both in and out of the gym.

However, she also said that she has learned to use her ADHD to her advantage, as it has given her a sense of focus and drive in her training and competition.

Biles has been open about her struggles with ADHD and has used her platform to raise awareness and advocate for a better understanding of the condition. She has encouraged others with ADHD to embrace their differences and to seek help if they need it.

Simone Biles' diagnosis with ADHD has not held her back in any way and has only made her more determined to succeed and inspire others to do the same.

These are just a few examples of successful public figures with ADHD who have been able to turn their ADHD into a positive force in their careers.

By seeing these examples, women with ADHD can gain inspiration and see that it is possible to overcome the challenges of ADHD and achieve great things.

Absolutely! The public figures and several others have been open about their struggles with ADHD, and their experiences can provide valuable lessons and encouragement to women with ADHD.

Here are some ways that women with ADHD can learn from these public figures:

Embrace your strengths: Many public figures with ADHD have found success by embracing their unique strengths and utilizing them in their careers. For example, Mandel has spoken about how his impulsiveness and creativity have helped him in his entertainment career.

Find ways to manage your symptoms: Many public figures have learned to manage their ADHD symptoms and maintain their success. For instance, actor and producer Channing Tatum has spoken about how he uses exercise and mindfulness practices to manage his ADHD.

Don't let ADHD define you: It's important for women with ADHD to remember that their condition does not define them. Public figures like musician Adam Levine and race car driver Dale Earnhardt Jr. have shared how they've overcome challenges related to ADHD and achieved great success in their lives.

Seek support: Having a supportive network of friends and family members can be incredibly helpful for managing ADHD. Actress and comedian Karla

Souza has spoken about the importance of having a supportive partner in her life.

By learning from these public figures and others, women with ADHD can gain insight and encouragement as they work towards living their best lives.

Chapter Ten: Managing ADHD as a modern woman

20 Essential Tips for Success

1. Women with ADHD must know their diagnosis and understand the symptoms.

2. It's important to have a support system and connect with others who have ADHD.

3. Regular exercise and healthy eating habits can help manage symptoms.

4. Women with ADHD should seek professional help, such as therapy or coaching.

5. Time management and organization skills can be developed with practice.

6. Medication can be an effective tool for managing symptoms, but it's important to find the right type and dosage.

7. Women with ADHD should take breaks and prioritize self-care.

8. Understanding triggers and stressors can help reduce symptoms.

9. Women with ADHD can benefit from developing a daily routine.

10. Embracing strengths and learning to work with weaknesses can lead to success and fulfillment.

11. Women with ADHD should not ignore their diagnosis or be ashamed of their symptoms.

12. It's not helpful to compare oneself to others and focus on limitations.

13. Avoiding professional help and support can lead to further challenges.

14. Substance abuse and unhealthy coping mechanisms can worsen symptoms.

15. Procrastination and disorganization can hinder success and productivity.

16. Ignoring treatment options, such as medication, can prevent symptom management.

17: Overloading oneself with too many responsibilities can lead to burnout.

18: Blaming others for challenges and not taking responsibility for one's actions can cause harm to relationships.

19. Women with ADHD should not dismiss their intuition and inner voice.

20. Giving up on personal goals and aspirations is not a solution to managing ADHD.

If you're a woman with ADHD always know that:

1. You have a unique perspective and approach to problem-solving.

2. You have the ability to think creatively and outside of the box.

3. You have a natural ability to multitask.

4. You have the ability to hyperfocus and get things done quickly.

5. You have a natural sense of adventure and excitement for life.

6. You have a strong sense of independence and don't follow the crowd.

7. You have a natural ability to see humor in situations.

8. You have a gift for making connections between seemingly unrelated things.

9. You have a passion for learning and personal growth.

10. You are resilient and don't give up easily.

11. You have a unique ability to see the beauty in the world.

12. You have a natural ability to see opportunities where others see obstacles.

13. You have a zest for life and are always up for trying new things.

14. You have a natural curiosity and desire to understand the world.

15. You have a strong sense of empathy and compassion for others.

16. You have a talent for adapting to change and handling unexpected situations.

17. You have a strong sense of self-awareness and introspection.

18. You have a natural ability to see the positive in negative situations.

19. You have a strong desire to make a positive impact on the world.

20. You have a talent for engaging and inspiring others.

21. You have a natural ability to think on your feet.

22. You have a talent for developing creative solutions to problems.

23. You have a passion for helping others and making a difference.

24. You have a natural talent for prioritizing and organizing tasks.

25. You have a unique ability to see the big picture and think long-term.

26. You have a natural ability to stay focused and motivated.

27. You have a strong sense of determination and drive.

28. You have a natural talent for leadership and guiding others.

29. You have a talent for building relationships and connecting with others.

30. You have a unique ability to see things from different angles.

31. You have a natural ability to stay calm under pressure.

32. You have a talent for taking calculated risks and stepping outside of your comfort zone.

33. You have a natural ability to think critically and analyze situations.

34. You have a talent for identifying patterns and finding solutions.

35. You have a strong desire to make the world a better place.

36. You have a talent for staying organized and focused even in chaotic situations.

37. You have a natural ability to see the potential in others and bring out their best.

38. You have a talent for overcoming obstacles and finding solutions to problems.

39. You have a natural ability to see the potential in yourself and work towards self-improvement.

40. You have a strong sense of self-confidence and belief in yourself.
41. You have a talent for adapting to new situations and learning quickly.

42. You have a natural ability to think outside of the box and come up with innovative solutions.

43. You have a strong sense of purpose and a clear vision for your life.

44. You have a natural talent for staying focused on your goals and working towards success.

45. You have a natural ability to prioritize and manage your time effectively.

46. You have a strong sense of self-motivation and drive to achieve your goals.

47. You have a natural talent for overcoming obstacles and persevering through challenges.

48. You have a strong sense of self-awareness and the ability to overcome.

In conclusion, ADHD and the modern woman is a subject that deserves our attention and understanding. Women with ADHD face unique challenges and obstacles in their daily lives, often feeling overwhelmed and undervalued. However, with the right strategies and support, they can thrive and lead fulfilling lives.

One key strategy for managing ADHD is to build a support system. This can include seeking out professional help from a therapist, joining a support group, or seeking guidance from friends and family. Additionally, medication can be an effective way to manage the symptoms of ADHD, but it is important to work closely with a doctor to determine the right approach.

Another key strategy is to develop coping mechanisms and routines that work for you. This may include creating a structured schedule, using a planner or task list, or taking regular breaks to refocus and recharge. It can also be helpful to identify triggers that lead to symptoms of ADHD, such as stress or lack of sleep, and finding ways to manage them.

Finally, it is important to cultivate a positive self-image and to recognize and value one's strengths and achievements. Women with ADHD often struggle with feelings of inadequacy, but it is important to remember that ADHD is not a reflection of intelligence or worth. By focusing on strengths and successes, women with ADHD can build confidence and resilience.

ADHD and the modern woman is a complex and often misunderstood subject, but with the right tools and support, women with

ADHD can lead fulfilling and productive lives.

Whether you are a woman with ADHD or a loved one, it is important to understand and support the unique challenges faced by those with this condition. With the right strategies, women with ADHD can overcome obstacles, reach their goals, and live the life they deserve.

Appreciation

Dear reader,

I hope that this book has been a valuable resource for you in your journey to better understand and manage ADHD in your life or that of a loved one.

As modern women, we face many demands and challenges, and navigating ADHD can feel overwhelming at times. However, by using the strategies and tools outlined in this book, I believe that you can find greater balance, peace, and fulfillment in your daily life.

I want to take this moment to thank you for taking the time to read through this book. Your commitment to understanding and improving your situation is a testament to your strength and determination. I am grateful for the opportunity to share my knowledge and experience with you, and I hope that you have found this book to be a supportive and empowering guide on your journey.

If you have found the information in this book to be helpful, I encourage you to continue exploring and learning more about ADHD. There are many resources available, both online and in your community, which can provide you with additional support and guidance. Remember to take care of yourself, prioritize self-compassion, and

don't be afraid to reach out for help when you need it.

Once again, thank you for choosing "ADHD and the Modern Woman: Strategies for Managing Life's Demands." I wish you all the best as you continue to navigate ADHD and build the life you deserve.

Sincerely,
Brenda Maye